# Electric Pressure Cooker Cookbook

50+ Foolproof Recipes that Cook for Themselves in your Instant Pot, Plus Tips and Tricks to Get the Best Result Every Single Time

**Maria Marshal**

# Table Of Contents

# BREAKFAST RECIPES

## Biscuits with Bacon Gravy

*(Ready in about 15 minutes | Servings 8)*

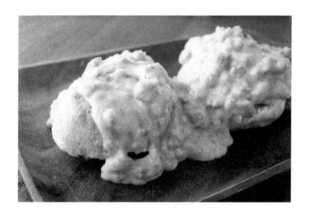

### *Ingredients*

1. 2 bacon strips, finely diced

1. 1 pound sausage

1. 1 teaspoon rosemary, chopped

1. 1 teaspoon dried thyme, chopped

1. 1/2 cup vegetable broth

1. 1/4 cup wheat flour

1. 1 ½ cups whole milk

1. 1/2 teaspoon salt

1. 1 teaspoon cracked black pepper

1. Prepared biscuits

## *Directions*

1. First of all, make the sauce. Set your pressure cooker to HIGH. Then, placebacon strips and sausage in the bottom of your cooker; sauté until they are browned, approximately 7 minutes.

2. Sprinkle with rosemary and thyme. Pour in vegetable broth. Now securely lock the lid and set on HIGH for about 5 minutes. Now release the cooker'spressure.

3. In a bowl or a measuring cup, whisk the flour and milk. Add this mixture tothe cooker; let simmer for 3 minutes, or until the juice has thickened.

4. Season with salt and black pepper. To serve, spoon the bacon gravy overprepared biscuits and enjoy.

# Cheese Spoon Bread

*(Ready in about 20 minutes | Servings 6)*

## Ingredients

1. 1 cup whole milk

1. 2 cups vegetable stock

1. 2/3 cup cornmeal

1. 1 cup baking mix

1. 1 cup sharp cheese, shredded

1. 2 eggs

1. 2 tablespoons butter, melted

1. 2 teaspoons sugar

1. 1/2 teaspoon black pepper

1. 1 teaspoon salt

1. 1/2 teaspoon onion powder

1. 1 teaspoon granulated garlic

## *Directions*

1. Brush the inside of the cooker with nonstick cooking spray.

2. In a bowl, combine all the above components. Now add this mixture to thepressure cooker. Securely lock the lid and set for 8 minutes on LOW.

3. Then, leave steam valve open. Set the cooker to "Brown" and let it cookapproximately 5 minutes. Turn off the heat and let stand for 5 minutesbefore serving.

# Super Creamy Potato Salad

*(Ready in about 20 minutes + chilling time | Servings 6)*

## *Ingredients*

1. 8 small-sized red potatoes, scrubbed

1. 1 cup water

1. 1 medium-sized onion, chopped

1. 1 carrot, chopped

1. 1 stalk celery, chopped

1. 1 teaspoon cayenne pepper

1. 1/2 teaspoon dried rosemary

1. 3/4 teaspoon sea salt

1. 1/4 teaspoon black pepper, freshly cracked

1. 3 whole hard-boiled eggs, chopped

1. 1/2 cup mayonnaise

1. 1 teaspoon apple cider vinegar

## Directions

1. Place potatoes together with water in your pressure cooker. Then, you should cook them on high pressure for about 3 minutes. Now let steamrelease for 2 to 3 minutes.

2. Now, quickly release the pressure in order to open pressure cooker. Allowthe potatoes to cool enough to handle. Peel and slice them. Place a single layer of potatoes in a bowl.

3. Alternate potato layers with onions, carrot, and celery layers. Sprinkle eachlayer with cayenne pepper, rosemary, salt, and freshly cracked black pepper. Top your salad with the eggs.

4. In a mixing bowl, mix together the mayonnaise and apple cider vinegar.Now fold this mayonnaise mixture into the vegetables. Allow the salad tochill in a refrigerator before serving. Serve chilled.

# Protein Lentil Salad

*(Ready in about 20 minutes | Servings 6)*

### Ingredients

1. 1 cup dried lentils, rinsed

1. 2 cups chicken broth

1. 1 bay leaf

1. 1 medium-sized carrot, diced

1. 1 medium-sized onion, finely diced

1. 2 tablespoons olive oil

1. 2 tablespoons white wine

1. 1 clove garlic, minced

1. 2 tablespoons fresh cilantro, chopped

1. 1/2 teaspoon dried basil

1. 3/4 teaspoon salt

1. 1/4 teaspoon pepper

## *Directions*

1. Add lentils, chicken broth, and bay leaf to the pressure cooker.

2. Securely lock the lid and then, set on HIGH for 8 minutes. Remove the lid;then, drain lentils and discard the bay leaf.

3. Combine prepared lentils with the remaining ingredients. Serve warm or atroom temperature.

# Apples and Pears in Strawberry Sauce

*(Ready in about 25 minutes | Servings 4)*

## Ingredients

1. 2 medium-sized pears, peeled, cored, and halved

1. 2 medium-sized apples, peeled, cored, and halved

1. 1 cup water

1. 1 pint strawberries

1. 1 vanilla bean, sliced lengthwise

1. 1/2 teaspoon grated nutmeg

1. 1/4 teaspoon ground cardamom

1. 1/2 cup light brown sugar

1. 1 tablespoon cornstarch

## Directions

1. Put all ingredients, except for brown sugar and cornstarch, into the pressure cooker. Now securely lock the pressure cooker's lid.

2. Set the cooker on LOW for 7 minutes. Then, remove pears and set aside.

3. Next, mash the strawberries with a heavy spoon. Combine the sugar andcornstarch with 1 tablespoon of water.

4. Now, set cooker to "Brown,"; stir in dissolved sugar-cornstarch mixture.Allow it to simmer for 3 to 5 minutes, or until strawberry sauce has thickened.

5. Divide the pears and apples among serving plates. Top with strawberrysauce, serve and enjoy.

# FAST SNACKS RECIPES
## Hummus with Pita Chips

*(Ready in about 1 hour | Servings 16)*

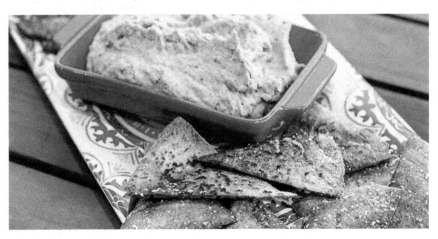

### *Ingredients*

1. 1 cup chickpeas

1. 2 teaspoons canola oil

1. 4 cups water

1. 1 tablespoon fresh cilantro

1. 1 teaspoon dried parsley

1. 2 cloves garlic, peeled and minced

1. 2 tablespoons tahini

1. 1/4 teaspoon dried spearmint

1. 3/4 teaspoon salt, to taste

1. 2 tablespoons lemon juice

1. 1/4 cup sesame oil

1. Pita chips, for garnish

### *Directions*

1. Add the chickpeas, canola oil, and 4 cups of water to your cooker. Cover and bring to HIGH pressure; maintain for 40 minutes. Then, allow pressureto release naturally.

2. Uncover, drain the chickpeas and cook on HIGH pressure for an additional10 minutes.

3. Add the prepared chickpeas to your food processor (or a blender). Now stirin cilantro, parsley, garlic, tahini, spearmint, salt, and lemon juice. Pulse until everything is well combined. Make sure to scrape down the sides ofthe food processor bowl.

4. Lastly, add the sesame oil with the machine running and pulse until it issmooth. Serve with pita chips and enjoy!

# Fastest-Ever Corn Cobs

*(Ready in about 10 minutes | Servings 6)*

## Ingredients

1. 3 cups water

1. 6 ears sweet corn cobs, halved

## Directions

1. Pour the water into your pressure cooker; insert the steamer basket.

2. Place the corn cobs in the steamer basket.

3. Seal the lid. Set the timer to 2 minutes under HIGH pressure. Run thecooker under cold water. Serve warm.

# Traditional Baba Ghanoush

*(Ready in about 15 minutes | Servings 16)*

## *Ingredients*

1. 1 tablespoon sesame oil

1. 1 large-sized eggplant, peeled and diced

1. 5 cloves garlic, finely minced

1. 1/2 cup water

1. 3 tablespoons fresh cilantro

1. 3/4 teaspoon salt

1. Cracked black pepper, to taste

1. 1 tablespoon lemon juice

1. 2 tablespoons tahini

1. 1 tablespoon olive oil

## *Directions*

1. Add the sesame oil to the pressure cooker; heat over medium heat. Stir in the eggplant. Sauté the eggplant until it is tender. Add the garlic; sauté for30 seconds more.

2. Pour in the water, and lock the lid. Bring to HIGH pressure; maintain pressure for 4 to 5 minutes. Then, quick-release the pressure, and uncover.

3. Add the eggplant mixture to a food processor along with the cilantro, salt,black pepper, lemon juice, and tahini. Process it, scraping down the sides ofthe container.

4. Add the olive oil and process until smooth. Transfer to a serving bowl.Serve with your favorite pita wedges or veggie sticks.

# Artichoke and Spinach Dip

*(Ready in about 15 minutes | Servings 12)*

## Ingredients
1. 2 cups canned artichoke hearts, coarsely chopped

1. 1 ½ cups frozen chopped spinach, thawed and well drained

1. 1/2 cup sour cream

1. 1/2 cup mayonnaise

1. 1 ½ cups mozzarella cheese, shredded

1. 1/2 teaspoon paprika

1. Sea salt and ground black pepper, to taste

## Directions

1. Combine all the ingredients together in a baking dish that fits in the pressure cooking pot. Cover it tightly with a foil. Make sure to prepare afoil sling.

2. Place the rack at the bottom of the cooker. Pour about 2 cups of water intothe cooker. Place the baking dish on the rack.

3. Seal the lid and select HIGH pressure for 10 minutes. After that, turn off thecooker; use a quick pressure release; then, carefully remove the lid.

4. Serve warm with tortilla chips if desired. Enjoy!

# Amazing Steamed Artichokes

*(Ready in about 10 minutes | Servings 6)*

### Ingredients

1. 3 medium artichokes

1. 1 medium-sized lemon, halved

1. 1 teaspoon yellow mustard

1. 3 tablespoons mayonnaise

1. 1/2 teaspoon cayenne pepper

1. Salt and ground black pepper, to taste

### Directions

1. Pour 1 cup of water into the pressure cooker. Now place the steamer basketin your cooker. Add the artichokes; drizzle with lemon.

2. Close the lid and turn the heat to HIGH; Cook for 10 minutes at highpressure.

3. Then, open the pressure cooker with the natural release method. Check forthe doneness. If it is not done, cook for an additional few minutes.

4. Then, make the sauce. In a mixing bowl, combine the mustard together withmayonnaise, cayenne pepper, salt, and black pepper. Serve with prepared artichokes. Serve warm.

# LUNCH RECIPES
## Meatball Soup with Noodles
*(Ready in about 20 minutes | Servings 6)*

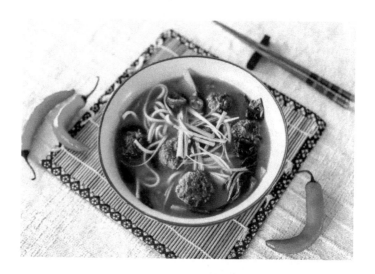

### *Ingredients*

1. 2 tablespoons canola oil

1. 1 onion, thinly sliced

1. 1 cup carrot, sliced

1. 6 cups vegetable broth

1. 1 (16-ounce) bag frozen Italian meatballs

1. 1 cup dried noodles

1. 2 cups spinach, torn into pieces

1. 1 tablespoon lemon juice

1. 2 cloves garlic, minced

1. Salt and ground black pepper, to taste

## *Directions*

1. First, heat the oil on HIGH until sizzling. Now sauté the onion and carrotfor about 5 minutes.

2. Add the rest of the above ingredients. Securely lock the lid and set for 5minutes on HIGH.

3. Taste and adjust the seasonings. Serve warm and enjoy!

# Creamy Cauliflower and Cheese Soup

*(Ready in about 10 minutes | Servings 6)*

## *Ingredients*

1. 2 tablespoons butter

1. 1 medium-sized leek, sliced

1. 1 small-sized head cauliflower, chopped

1. 2-3 baby carrots, trimmed and chopped

1. 4 cups chicken broth

1. 1 bay leaf

1. 1/2 teaspoon cayenne pepper

1. 1 teaspoon granulated garlic

1. 1 cup heavy cream

1. 1 cup sharp cheese, shredded

1. Salt and cracked black pepper, to taste

# Directions

1. Warm the butter in your cooker until sizzling. Then, sauté the leeks untiltranslucent, or for about 5 minutes.

2. Add the cauliflower, carrots, chicken broth, 1 bay leaf, cayenne pepper, andgranulated garlic. Now lock the pressure cooker's lid; set for 4 minutes onHIGH. Then, release the cooker's pressure.

3. Stir in heavy cream and shredded sharp cheese; season with salt and blackpepper. Serve.

# Mom's Corn Chowder

*(Ready in about 25 minutes | Servings 6)*

### Ingredients

1. 1 tablespoon olive oil

1. 1 shallot, diced

1. 2 cloves garlic, peeled and minced

1. 1 carrot, chopped

1. 1 celery stalk, chopped

1. 5 cups fresh corn kernels, cut off the cob

1. 3 cups vegetable broth

1. 3⁄4 teaspoon salt

1. 1/4 teaspoon ground black pepper

1. 1 (12-ounce) can evaporated milk

1. 2 tablespoons cornstarch

1. 3 tablespoons margarine

## *Directions*

1. In your pressure cooker, heat olive oil over HIGH setting. Now, sauté theshallot and garlic for 4 to 5 minutes.

2. Add carrot, celery, corn kernels, vegetable broth, salt, and ground black pepper; securely lock the lid, and cook the soup for 6 minutes on HIGH.

3. In a small bowl, whisk together the milk and cornstarch; stir the mixture into your soup. Stir in the margarine. Let simmer for 2 to 3 minutes, or untilthe soup has thickened. Serve warm with the croutons if desired.

# Chunky Butternut Bean Soup

*(Ready in about 1 hour | Servings 6)*

## Ingredients

1. 2 tablespoons olive oil

1. 1 medium-sized leek, chopped

1. 2 carrots, chopped medium

1. 2 celery stalks, chopped

1. 3 sprigs fresh thyme

1. 16 ounces dried beans

1. 9 cups vegetables broth

1. Sea salt and black pepper, to taste

1. 1/2 teaspoon dried dill weed

1. 1/2 teaspoon dried rosemary, chopped

1. 2 cups butternut squash, diced

1. 1/2 cup sour cream

## Directions

1. Warm olive oil in your pressure cooker; sauté leek, carrot, and celery untilthey are softened.

2. Add the thyme, beans, broth, salt, and black pepper. Cook for 35 minuteson HIGH.

3. Using cold water method, open the cooker's lid; add dill, rosemary, andbutternut squash. Cover and cook for 10 more minutes.

4. Serve with a dollop of sour cream. Enjoy!

# Cheesy Potato and Spinach Soup

*(Ready in about 20 minutes | Servings 6)*

## *Ingredients*

1. 1⁄4 cup vegetable oil

1. 6 white onions, white part only, sliced

1. 1 red bell pepper, seeded and chopped

1. 2 celery stalks, chopped

1. 1⁄2 cup rice

1. 3 potatoes, peeled and diced

1. 5 cups vegetable stock

1. 3/4 teaspoon sea salt

1. 1⁄4 teaspoon ground black pepper

1. 2 tablespoons white wine

1. 3 tablespoons tomato paste

1. 1 ½ cups fresh spinach, torn into large pieces

1. 1⁄2 cup Monterey Jack cheese, grated

## Directions

1. In a pressure cooker, warm vegetable oil. Add onions, bell pepper, andcelery; sauté for about 2 minutes.

2. Stir in rice and potatoes. Continue cooking an additional minute.

3. Add vegetable stock, salt, black pepper, wine, and tomato paste. Stir well tocombine.

4. Seal the lid and cook on high pressure. Now reduce the heat to maintainpressure, and cook for 4 minutes. Uncover and divide among soup bowls.Garnish with grated cheese and serve warm.

# DINNER RECIPES
## Yummy Vegan Gumbo
*(Ready in about 2 hours | Servings 6)*

### Ingredients

1. 1/2 cup canola oil

1. 1/2 cup all-purpose flour

1. 1 onion, diced

1. 1 red bell pepper, diced

1. 1 carrot, diced

1. 1 stalk celery, diced

1. 4 cloves garlic, minced

1. 2 cups vegetable broth

1. 4 cups water

1. 1 tablespoon Vegan Worcestershire sauce

1. 1 (16-ounce) package frozen chopped okra

1. 2 bay leaves

1. Sea salt and black pepper, to taste

1. 1 pound vegan chicken, chopped

1. 1/2 cup parsley, chopped

1. 6 cups hot cooked rice

### Directions

1. Warm canola oil over medium heat in your pressure cooker. To make the roux: add the flour and cook, stirring frequently, until your roux gets a rich brown color, or for about 25 minutes.

2. Add the onion, bell pepper, carrot, celery, and garlic to the roux; continue to sauté for 5 minutes. Add the broth and water, bringing to a boil over HIGH heat for 20 minutes.

3. Add the rest of the above ingredients, except for rice. Cover, bring to LOW pressure and maintain for 1 hour 10 minutes. Afterwards, allow pressure to release naturally.

4. Serve over prepared rice and enjoy!

# Barley and Chickpea Stew

*(Ready in about 20 minutes | Servings 4)*

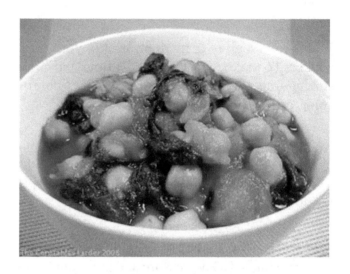

## *Ingredients*

1. 1 cup barley

1. 1 cup dry chickpeas, soaked

1. 2 tablespoons olive oil, divided

1. 2 cloves garlic, pressed

1. 1 onion, diced

1. 2 carrots, diced

1. 1 parsnip, chopped

1. 2 celery stalks, diced

1. 1/2 head red cabbage, shredded

1. 4 cups water

1. 1 teaspoon sea salt

1. 1/2 teaspoon ground black pepper

1. 1/2 teaspoon cayenne pepper

## *Directions*

1. Simply throw all of the above ingredients in the pressure cooker. Close andlock the lid.

2. Turn the heat to HIGH and cook your stew for 15 minutes at HIGHpressure.

3. Open with a natural release method. Release the rest of the pressure withthe cooker's valve.

4. Season to taste and serve right away!

# Asian-Style Tofu Stew

*(Ready in about 15 minutes | Servings 4)*

### Ingredients

1. 2 tablespoons sesame oil

1. 1 small-sized onion, sliced

1. 2 cloves garlic, minced

1. 1 cup broccoli, chopped into florets

1. 1 cup mushrooms, sliced

1. 12 ounces soft silken tofu, drained and cubed

1. 1 tablespoon red pepper, crushed

1. 1 teaspoon tamari sauce

1. 3 cups vegetable stock

1. Fresh chives, for garnish

### Directions

1. Warm the sesame oil over medium heat in your pressure cooker. Then, sauté the onion and garlic for 3 to 4 minutes.

2. Add the rest of your ingredients, except for chives, to the pressure cooker.Cover with the lid; bring to LOW pressure and maintain for 5 minutes. Remove from heat and allow pressure to release naturally.

3. Remove the lid and serve in individual bowls. Sprinkle with chives. Enjoy!

# Beef and
# Mushroom Stew

*(Ready in about 35 minutes | Servings 8)*

## Ingredients

1. 1 (3-pound) chuck roast, cut into bite-sized pieces

1. 2 (4-ounce) cans mushrooms, drained and sliced

1. 2 (10 3/4-ounce) cans cream of mushroom soup

1. 2 cups water

1. 1 tablespoon Worcestershire sauce

1. 3 (24-ounce) bags frozen vegetables, thawed

1. Salt and freshly ground black pepper, to taste

1. 1 teaspoon red pepper flakes, crushed

## Directions

1. Add chuck roast, mushroom, mushroom soup, water, and Worcestershiresauce to the pressure cooker.

2. Then, bring to LOW pressure; maintain pressure for 30 minutes. Stir in frozen vegetables. Bring to a simmer and maintain pressure for 5 minutes.

3. Sprinkle with salt, black pepper, and red pepper. Taste for seasoning andserve warm.

# Veggies in Lime-Butter Sauce

*(Ready in about 10 minutes | Servings 6)*

## Ingredients

1. 2 cups cauliflower florets

1. 2 cups broccoli florets

1. 1/2 teaspoon salt

1. 1/2 teaspoon black pepper

1. 1/2 teaspoon dried dill weed

1. 1 cup water

1. 4 tablespoons butter

1. 1 tablespoon lime juice

1. 1/2 teaspoon yellow mustard

## Directions

1. Put the cauliflower, broccoli, salt, black pepper, dried dill, and water into your pressure cooker. Cover and bring to LOW pressure; maintain pressure for 2 to 3 minutes.
2. Turn off the heat; quick-release the pressure; remove the cooker's lid.
3. To make the sauce: whisk together the butter, lime juice, and yellow mustard. Drizzle the sauce over the cooked cauliflower and broccoli. Serve.

# DESSERT RECIPES
## A-Number-1 Banana Cake

*(Ready in about 40 minutes | Servings 12)*

### Ingredients

1. 1 ½ cups all-purpose flour

1. 1/2 teaspoon baking soda

1. 1 teaspoon baking powder

1. 1 teaspoon vanilla essence

1. 1 cup granulated sugar

1. A pinch of salt

1. A dash of cinnamon

1. 2 medium-sized ripe bananas, mashed

1. 1/2 cup butter, melted

1. 1 cup soymilk

### Directions

1. In a medium-sized bowl, combine together the flour, baking soda, bakingpowder, vanilla essence, sugar, and salt.

2. Add cinnamon and mashed bananas. Slowly stir in the butter and thesoymilk. Gently stir until everything is well incorporated.

3. Pour the batter into a round pan. Lay the pan in the pressure cooker. Coverand cook the cake for 30 minutes over LOW heat.

4. Afterwards, carefully remove the cake from the pan. Serve at roomtemperature.

# Orange Cornmeal Cake

*(Ready in about 20 minutes | Servings 6)*

## *Ingredients*

1. 2 cups milk

1. 1/4 cup light brown sugar

1. 1 teaspoon orange zest, grated

1. 1/2 cup fine yellow cornmeal

1. 2 large eggs

1. 2 tablespoons butter, softened

1. 2 tablespoons orange marmalade

1. 1/2 teaspoon vanilla extract

1. 1 cup water

## *Directions*

1. To make the batter: Bring milk to a simmer over
   MEDIUM heat. Stir in the sugar and continue to simmer
   for about 2 minutes.

2. Whisk in the orange zest and yellow cornmeal.
   Simmer for 2 minuteslonger, stirring
   continuously.

3. Remove from the heat. In a separate mixing bowl, whisk together the eggs,softened butter, orange marmalade, and vanilla extract. Stir the egg mixture into the cornmeal mixture.

4. Coat a heatproof glass dish with non-stick cooking spray. Add preparedcake batter.

5. Pour 1 cup of water into the pressure cooker; now place a rack in your cooker. Place the dish on the rack. Cook on LOW pressure for 12 minutes.Allow to sit for a few minutes before removing from the dish.

# Old-Fashioned Chocolate Cake

*(Ready in about 45 minutes | Servings 12)*

## Ingredients

1.  1 ½ cups all-purpose flour

1.  4 tablespoons cocoa powder

1.  1/4 teaspoon grated nutmeg

1.  1 teaspoon cinnamon

1.  1 tablespoon maple syrup

1.  1/2 teaspoon almond extract

1.  A pinch of salt

1.  1/2 teaspoon baking powder

1.  1/2 teaspoon baking soda

1.  2 eggs, beaten

1.  4 tablespoons butter, melted

1.  1 cup whole milk

1.  2 cups hot water

## Directions

1. In a mixing bowl, combine together the flour, cocoa powder, nutmeg, cinnamon, maple syrup, almond extract, salt, baking powder, and bakingsoda.

2. In another bowl, beat the eggs. Add to the dry flour mixture. Then, stir inthe melted butter and the milk. Stir to combine well. Replace the cake mixture to a round cake pan.

3. Add the rack to the pressure cooker; pour in the water. Place the cake pan on the rack. Bring to HIGH pressure; then reduce to LOW and cook for 30minutes. Let the cake sit for 10 minutes; carefully remove your cake from the pan. Cut into wedges and serve.

# Coconut Rice Pudding with Raisins

*(Ready in about 30 minutes | Servings 6)*

### Ingredients

1. 1 ½ cups white rice, rinsed and drained

1. 1 (14-ounce) can coconut milk

1. 1 cup water

1. 2 cups whole milk

1. 1/2 cup granulated sugar

1. 1/4 teaspoon cardamom

1. 1/4 teaspoon nutmeg, freshly grated

1. 1 teaspoons ground cinnamon

1. A pinch of salt

1. 1 cup golden raisins

### Directions

1. Add rice, coconut milk, water, milk, sugar, cardamom, nutmeg, cinnamon,and salt to your pressure cooker. Now cook over medium-high heat, bringing to a gentle boil.

2. Lock the lid into place; cook on LOW pressure for 15 minutes.

3. Afterwards, remove the lid according to manufacturer's directions. Stir ingolden raisins. Allow the pudding to stand for about 15 minutes. Serve.

# Vegan Chocolate Cake

*(Ready in about 45 minutes | Servings 12)*

## Ingredients

1. 1 ½ cups all-purpose flour

1. 4 tablespoons cocoa powder

1. 1 teaspoon cinnamon

1. 1/2 teaspoon cardamom

1. 1 teaspoon anise

1. 1 tablespoon maple syrup

1. 1/2 teaspoon vanilla extract

1. A pinch of salt

1. 1 teaspoon baking powder

1. 2 ripe bananas

1. 4 tablespoons vegan margarine, melted

1. 1 cup almond milk

1. 2 cups hot water

## Directions

1. In a bowl, combine together the flour, cocoa powder, cinnamon, cardamom,anise seed maple syrup, vanilla, salt, and baking powder. In a separate mixing bowl, whisk the bananas, together with vegan margarine, and almond milk.

2. Add banana mixture to the dry flour mixture; stir to combine well. Replacethe batter to a round cake pan.

3. Place the rack in your pressure cooker; pour hot water into the bottom of your cooker. Place the pan on the rack. Now cook for 30 minutes on LOW.Allow your cake to rest at least 10 minutes. Serve.

# INSTANT POT

# BREAKFAST RECIPES
## Rice Pudding with Zante Currants
*(Ready in about 30 minutes | Servings 6)*

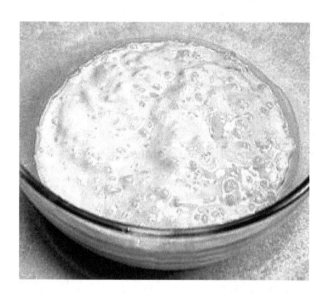

**Ingredients**

1. 1 ½ cups rice

1. 1/2 cup sugar

1. 1 tablespoon honey

1. A pinch of sea salt

1. 5 cups milk

1. 2 whole eggs

1. 1 cup half and half

1. 1 cup Zante currants

1. 1/2 teaspoon freshly grated nutmeg

## *Directions*

1. In the inner pot, combine together the rice, sugar, honey, salt, and milk. Choose the "Sauté" button; bring to a boil. Stir in order to dissolve thesugar.

2. Cover your instant pot. Turn to the stream release to "SEALING" position. Press the "Rice" button. After about 15 minutes perform the quick pressure release

3. In the meantime, whisk the eggs and half and half in a mixing bowl.

4. Remove the lid from the pot. Stir in the egg mixture. Now add Zante currants and grated nutmeg. Press the "Sauté". Cook, uncovered, until it starts to boil. Then, turn off the cooker.

5. Serve right away. If you want to serve chilled, it is good to know that thepudding will thicken as it cools. Enjoy!

# Cinnamon Fig Bread Pudding

*(Ready in about 45 minutes | Servings 4)*

## Ingredients

1. 6 slices of cinnamon bread, torn into pieces

1. 3 whole eggs

1. 3 cups milk

1. 1/2 teaspoon vanilla paste

1. 1/4 teaspoon kosher salt

1. 1/2 cup sugar

1. 1 tablespoon honey

1. 1/2 teaspoon cinnamon powder

1. 1 cup dried figs, chopped

## Directions

1. Coat a 5 cup bowl with non-stick cooking spray (butter flavor). Simply throw cinnamon bread pieces into the bowl.

2. In a separate bowl, mix all the remaining ingredients, except for figs. Pour this custard mixture over bread pieces. Scatter chopped dried figs over the top. Allow to sit for about 15 minutes to let bread pieces absorb the custardmixture.

58

3. Cover bowl tightly with a piece of buttered foil.

4. Put a steaming rack into the inner pot; pour in two cups of water.

5. Lock the cooker's lid. Use "Manual" setting on HIGH; cook for 25 minutes.Lastly, use a natural release for about 15 minutes.

# Vegan Summer Oatmeal

*(Ready in about 15 minutes | Servings 2)*

## Ingredients

1. 2 peaches, pitted and diced

1. 2 apricots, pitted and halved

1. 1 cup steel-cut oats

1. 1 cup almond milk

1. 1 teaspoon vanilla paste

1. 1/2 teaspoon cinnamon powder

1. 2 cups water

## Directions

1. Simply throw everything in the inner pot.

2. Now press "Manual"/ "Adjust"; set for 3 minutes.

3. Use 10 minutes natural release. Eat warm.

# Apricot Oats with Currants

*(Ready in about 15 minutes | Servings 2)*

## Ingredients

1. 1 cup steel-cut oats

1. 1 cup soy milk

1. 2 cups water

1. 1 tablespoon raw almond butter

1. 1 teaspoon ground flax seeds

1. 1/2 teaspoon cinnamon

1. 1/2 cup fresh apricot, chopped

1. 1/4 cup dried currants

## Directions

1. Add all the above ingredients to the inner pot of your Instant Pot.

2. Now press "Manual"/ "Adjust". Set for 3 minutes.

3. Lastly, perform natural release method.

# Easy Hard Boiled Eggs

*(Ready in about 10 minutes | Servings 2)*

## *Ingredients*

1.  1 cup water

1. 4 eggs

1.  Salt and freshly cracked black pepper, to taste

## *Directions*

1.  Pour the water into the pot; now position a steamer basket atop the rack.

2.  Place the eggs in the steamer basket, using canning lids to hold the eggs.

3.  Close the lid. Press "STEAM" setting; adjust time to 5 minutes. Lastly, quick release the steam valve. Then, transfer the eggs to a cold water forabout 2 minutes.

4.  Peel your eggs and season with salt and black pepper. Enjoy!

# LUNCH RECIPES
## Tomato Cabbage Rolls
*(Ready in about 1 hour | Servings 6)*

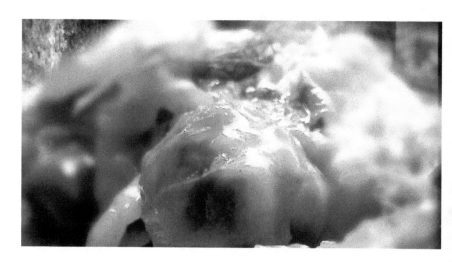

### *Ingredients*

1. 3 cloves garlic, minced

1. 1/2 cup onions chopped

1. 1 pound ground beef

1. 1 ½ cups rice

1. 2 (6.5-ounce) cans tomato sauce

1. 1 teaspoon cayenne pepper

1. Sea salt, to taste

1. 8 large cabbage leaves, blanched

1. Black peppercorns, to taste

1. 2 (10-ounce) cans diced tomatoes

### *Directions*

1. Combine the garlic, onion, beef, rice, tomato sauce, cayenne pepper, andsalt in a mixing bowl; mix until everything is well combined.

2. Divide the meat mixture among softened cabbage leaves. Roll the cabbageleaves up to form logs.

3. Place the rolls in a cooker. Add peppercorns and diced tomatoes.

4. Then, seal the lid of the cooker. Now cook for 1 hour under LOW pressure.Use the quick-release function. Serve warm.

# Juicy BBQ Pork

*(Ready in about 1 hour | Servings 8)*

### Ingredients

1.  8 pounds pork butt roast

1.  1 teaspoon garlic powder

1.  1 teaspoon cayenne pepper

1.  Sea salt and freshly ground black pepper, to taste

1.  2 (12-ounce) bottles BBQ sauce

### Directions

1.  Generously season the pork with garlic powder, cayenne pepper, salt, andblack pepper; place seasoned pork roast in your Instant Pot. Fill with enough water to cover the meat.

2.  Close the lid and bring up to 15 pounds of pressure. Cook on HIGHpressure for 1 hour.

3.  Reserve about 2 cups of pot juices. Shred the pork with two forks and mix with BBQ sauce, adding reserved juice. Serve warm over mashed potatoes.

# Herbed Pot Roast

*(Ready in about 35 minutes | Servings 8)*

## *Ingredients*

1. 3 pounds chuck roast

1. Salt and ground black pepper, to taste

1. 2 tablespoons canola oil

1. 1 onion, thinly sliced

1. 1 parsnip, peeled and thinly sliced

1. 1 carrot, peeled and thinly sliced

1. 1 celery stalk, thinly sliced

1. 8 red potatoes

1. 1 tablespoon tomato paste

1. 1 1/3 cups beef stock

1. 1 sprig thyme

1. 1 sprig rosemary

1. 4 cloves garlic, peeled and minced

1. 1/4 cup red wine

## *Directions*

1. Season the chuck roast with salt and ground black pepper.

2. Place the inner pot in your cooker. Place canola oil in the inner pot. Pressthe "MEAT" button. Sear the beef on all sides. Reserve the beef.

3. Add the vegetables to the inner pot and cook for about 3 minutes. Add thebeef back to the pot, along with the rest of the ingredients.

4. Place the lid on. Press the "WARM" button. Cook for 25 minutes. Carefullyremove the lid. Serve.

# Chicken Curry
# Soup

*(Ready in about 20 minutes | Servings 4)*

## *Ingredients*

1. 1 can coconut milk

1. 3 cups water

1. 1 teaspoon ground ginger

1. 1 teaspoon curry powder

1. 6 ounces frozen carrots

1. 6 ounces sugar snap peas

1. 6 ounces frozen okra

1. 1 medium-sized chicken breast, chopped

## *Directions*

1. Throw all ingredients into your Instant Pot.

2. Choose "Soup" setting. Serve hot and enjoy!

# Red Cabbage with Apples

*(Ready in about 35 minutes | Servings 4)*

## *Ingredients*

1. 2 tablespoons bacon fat

1. 1 onion, diced

1. 2 tart apples, peeled, cored and diced

1. 1 head red cabbage, shredded and stems removed

1. 1/4 red apple cider vinegar

1. 1 cup dry red wine

1. 1 cup beef stock

1. 1/2 teaspoon ground black pepper

1. 1/2 teaspoon dried thyme

1. 1 teaspoon sea salt

1. 1/2 teaspoon ground cloves

1. 3 tablespoons brown sugar, light or dark

1. 2 tablespoons all-purpose flour

1. 1 tablespoon cornstarch dissolved in 3 tablespoons dry red wine

## Directions

1. Set Instant Pot to "SAUTE". Warm bacon fat until it is completely melted.Then, sauté the onion and apples until soft, or approximately 10 minutes.Hit "Cancel" function.

2. Add the cabbage, apple cider vinegar, red wine, stock, ground black pepper,thyme, sea salt, ground cloves, and brown sugar.

3. Dust with flour; gently stir to combine. Select "Manual" and cook 8 to 10minutes. Perform a quick-release for 10 minutes.

4. Next, push "Sauté" and set to More. Bring to a boil; add prepared cornstarch slurry. Allow it to boil for about 5 minutes, or until cookingliquids are thickened. Serve warm.

# DINNER RECIPES
## Rice with Pineapple and Cauliflower
*(Ready in about 30 minutes | Servings 6)*

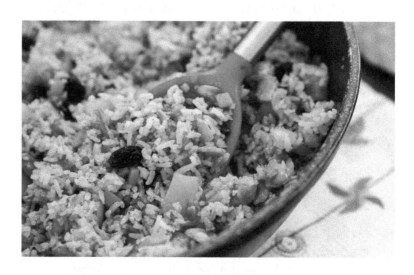

### *Ingredients*

1. 2 cups rice

1. 1/2 pineapple, cut into chunks

1. 1 broccoli, minced

1. 2 teaspoons olive oil

1. 1 teaspoon salt

1. 1/4 teaspoon white pepper

## Directions

1. Pour the water to the level 2 mark on the inner pot of your cooker.

2. Put the ingredients into the cooker. Choose the "Rice" button.

3. Serve warm, sprinkled with fresh parsley.

# Penne with Sausage and Tomato Sauce

*(Ready in about 20 minutes | Servings 6)*

## Ingredients

1. 1 cup bacon

1. 1 pound sausage meat

1. 1 shallot, finely chopped

1. 2 cloves garlic, minced

1. 2 cups tomato purée

1. Salt to taste

1. 1 pound pasta penne pasta

1. 1 teaspoon dried basil

1. 1 teaspoon dried oregano

1. 1/4 cup Parmesan cheese, grated

## Directions

1. Set the cooker on "Sauté". Cook the bacon for about 4 minutes. Now brownsausage until it's thoroughly cooked.

74

2. Add the shallot and garlic; sauté them for 4 minutes or until tender. Add therest of the ingredients, except for Parmesan cheese.

3. Choose "Manual", and LOW pressure for 5 minutes. Stir in Parmesancheese and serve right away. Bon appétit!

# Instant Pot Slow Cooker Meatloaf

*(Ready in about 8 hours | Servings 10)*

### Ingredients

For the Meatloaf:

1. Non-stick cooking spray

1. 1 pounds ground meat

1. 1 onion, finely chopped

1. 1 large-sized egg

1. 1 cup rice, cooked

1. 1 can drained mushrooms

1. 1 teaspoon onion powder

1. 1 teaspoon garlic powder

1. 1 cup milk

1. Salt and ground black pepper, to taste

1. 1 teaspoon dried thymeFor the Topping:

1. 1 tablespoon brown sugar

1. 3/4 cup ketchup

## Directions

1. Lightly oil an inner pot with non-stick cooking spray. Mix all ingredientsfor the meatloaf.

2. Shape the mixture into a round loaf; transfer it to the pot. Then, mix theingredients for the topping. Place the topping over the meatloaf.

3. Close and lock the cooker's lid. Choose the "Slow Cook" key and cook onLOW for 6 to 8 hours. Enjoy!

# Old-Fashioned Pork Belly

*(Ready in about 35 minutes | Servings 6)*

## Ingredients

1. 2 pounds pork belly, sliced

1. 1/2 cup soy sauce

1. 1 tablespoon sugar

1. 3 tablespoons cooking wine

1. 4-star anise

1. 2 cups water

1. 4 slices fresh ginger

1. 1 sweet onion, peeled and chopped

1. 6 cloves garlic, sliced

## Directions

1. Heat "Sauté"; then, sear pork belly on both sides. Add the remaining ingredients.

2. Press "Meat" key and cook for 30 minutes or so, until your meat are almostfalling apart. Serve right away!

# Friday Night Lasagna

*(Ready in about 30 minutes | Servings 6)*

## Ingredients

1. Non-stick cooking spray

1. 1 package dry lasagna noodles

1. 1 jar pasta sauce of choice

1. 1 ½ cups cream cheese

1. 1 cup mushrooms, thinly sliced

1. 1 teaspoon sea salt

1. 1/4 teaspoon ground black pepper

1. 1/4 teaspoon cayenne pepper

1. 1/2 teaspoon red pepper flakes

1. 1 teaspoon dried basil

1. 1/2 teaspoon dried rosemary

1. 1 teaspoon dried oregano

### *Directions*

1. Coat a spring-form pan with cooking spray.

2. Arrange lasagna noodles in the bottom of the pan. Then, spread the pastasauce. Lay your cream cheese.

3. Top with sliced fresh mushrooms. Sprinkle with some spices and herbs. Repeat the layers until you run out of ingredients. Cover with a piece of analuminum foil.

4. Next, place the trivet in the bottom of Instant Pot. Pour in 1 ½ cups water.Cook for 20 minutes under HIGH pressure.

5. Allow your lasagna to rest for about 10 minutes before removing from thepan.

# FAST SNACKS
## Roast Fingerling Potatoes
*(Ready in about 30 minutes | Servings 6)*

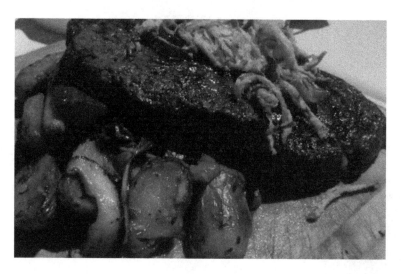

### *Ingredients*

1. 4 tablespoons canola oil

1. 2 pounds fingerling potatoes

1. 1 sprig thyme

1. 1 sprig rosemary

1. 1/2 teaspoon dried dill weed

1. 3 garlic cloves, with outer skin

1. 1 cup vegetable stock

1. Sea salt and ground black pepper, to your liking

## *Directions*

1. Use "Sauté" mode to pre-heat the cooker. Warm canola oil; when the oil ishot, stir in the potatoes, thyme, rosemary, dill, and garlic.

2. Cook the potatoes, turning occasionally, for about 10 minutes. Now piercein the middle of each potato with a sharp knife. Add vegetable stock, saltand black pepper to taste.

3. Choose "Manual" mode and cook for 11 minutes. Afterwards, use quickpressure release. Peel the garlic cloves and smash them. Taste, adjust theseasonings and serve.

# Saucy Turkey Wings

*(Ready in about 35 minutes | Servings 4)*

## Ingredients

1. 4 tablespoons butter, at room temperature

1. 4 turkey wings

1. Salt and ground black pepper, to your liking

1. 1 teaspoon cayenne pepper

1. 1 onion, sliced into rings

1. 1 ½ cups cranberries

1. 1/2 cup orange juice

1. 1 ½ cups vegetable stock

## Directions

1. Use "Sauté" setting and melt the butter. Brown your turkey wings on allsides. Season with salt, black pepper, and cayenne pepper.

2. Now add the onion rings and cranberries. Pour the orange juice and vegetable stock over all. Close the cooker's lid. Press "Manual" and choose20 minutes pressure cooking time.

3. Afterwards, preheat a broiler. Cook the wings under the broiler for about 5minutes.

4. While the wings are broiling, press "Sauté" button and cook the sauce uncovered in order to reduce the liquid content. Spoon the sauce over thewings and serve.

# Healthy Potato Snack

*(Ready in about 15 minutes | Servings 6)*

## Ingredients

1. 1/4 cup ghee

1. 1 ½ pounds russet potatoes, cut into wedges

1. Sea salt ground black pepper, to your liking

1. 1/2 teaspoon cayenne pepper

1. 1 teaspoon onion powder

1. 1 teaspoon cumin powder

1. 1/4 teaspoon allspice

1. 1 cup vegetable or chicken broth

## Directions

1. Choose "Sauté" mode and add ghee until it is warmed. Stir in the potatoes;cook for about 8 minutes.

2. Add the rest of the ingredients. Secure the lid, and press the "Manual" key.Cook for 7 minutes. Transfer to a serving platter and serve.

# Saucy Chicken Wings

*(Ready in about 15 minutes | Servings 8)*

## Ingredients

1. 1 tablespoon butter

1. 3/4 cup hot sauce

1. 4 pounds chicken wings, frozen

## Directions

1. Pour the butter and hot sauce into the inner pot of your Instant Pot. Add thewings.

2. Place the lid on cooker, and lock the lid. Press the "SOUP" button.

3. Serve with your favorite dipping sauce.

# Beets with Pine Nuts

*(Ready in about 25 minutes | Servings 8)*

### Ingredients

1. 2 ½ cups water

1. 2 pounds beets

1. 2 tablespoons cider vinegar

1. 2 teaspoons brown sugar

1. Sea salt and freshly ground black pepper, to your liking

1. 2 tablespoons extra-virgin olive oil

1. 2 tablespoons pine nuts, finely chopped

### Directions

1. Add the water and beets to your inner pot of the Instant Pot. Close lidsecurely.

2. Choose "Manual" and cook for 25 minutes. Remove lid. Drain and rinse beets; rub off skins. Cut your beets into wedges. Transfer to a serving bowl.

3. In a mixing bowl, combine vinegar, brown sugar, salt, black pepper, andolive oil. Drizzle the mixture over prepared beets; toss to combine. Scatterpine nuts over all and serve.

# DESSERT RECIPES
## Old-Fashioned Coconut Custard

*(Ready in about 35 minutes | Servings 8)*

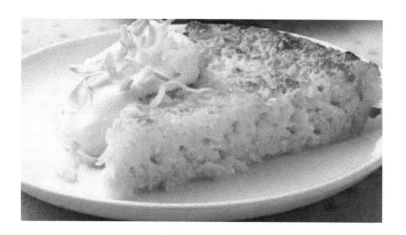

### *Ingredients*

1. 2 (14-ounce) cans coconut milk

1. 1 cup whole milk

1. 3 egg yolks

1. 3 whole eggs

1. 1 teaspoon pure vanilla extract

1. 2 cups water

## *Directions*

1. Pour coconut milk and whole milk into a saucepan; bring to a boil over highheat.

2. In another bowl, whisk the egg yolks with whole eggs. Now add 2 tablespoons of the warm milk mixture to the whisked eggs; add vanilla andmix until well combined.

3. Reduce the heat. Transfer the mixture to the simmering milk and stir. Continue simmering for about 4 minutes, stirring frequently.

4. Next, lightly grease a 6-cup soufflé pan; divide prepared egg-milk mixtureamong cups. Cover with an aluminum foil.

5. Pour the water into the cooker. Place a wire rack in your cooker; place thesoufflé dish on the rack. Cook for 30 minutes. Serve chilled.

# Classic Apple Crisp

*(Ready in about 15 minutes | Servings 6)*

## *Ingredients*

1. 4 apples, cored, peeled and sliced

1. 1 tablespoon fresh lemon juice

1. 1/2 cup old-fashioned oats

1. 1/4 cup flour

1. 1/4 cup brown sugar

1. 1 teaspoon vanilla essence

1. 1/2 teaspoon grated nutmeg

1. 1 teaspoon cinnamon powder

1. A pinch of sea salt

1. 4 tablespoons butter

1. 1 cup warm water

## *Directions*

1. First, sprinkle apples with lemon juice. In another
   bowl, combine oats, flour, sugar, vanilla, nutmeg,
   cinnamon powder, salt, and butter. Lay slicedapples in a
   baking dish. Place oat crisp mixture over it.

2. Cover baking dish with an aluminum foil. Pour water into the inner pot of the Instant Pot. Place trivet in the pot. Place the baking dish on trivet.

3. Now lock the lid and press the "BEANS" key; set the timer for 15 minutes. When the steam is completely released, remove the cooker's lid.

4. Remove the foil and let the dessert rest for several minutes. Enjoy!

# Bread Pudding with Golden Raisins

*(Ready in about 35 minutes | Servings 6)*

### Ingredients

1. 6 slices bread, torn into bite-sized pieces

1. 3 cups of milk

1. 3 eggs

1. 1 teaspoon vanilla

1. A pinch of salt

1. 1/4 cup sugar

1. 1 tablespoon honey

1. 1/4 teaspoon grated nutmeg

1. Golden raisins, to your liking

### Directions

1. Butter 5 cup bowl. Throw bread pieces into the bowl.

2. Then make the custard. In a mixing bowl, combine the milk, eggs, vanilla,salt, sugar, honey, and nutmeg.

3. Pour custard mixture over bread pieces. Now let bread pieces absorb egg-milk mixture. Scatter golden raisins over the top. Cover tightly with a foilthat has been greased.

4. Lay steaming rack in the inner pot. Pour in 2 cups water. Lock the cooker's lid.

5. Choose "Manual" setting on HIGH; set the timer for 25 minutes. Afterwards, perform a natural pressure release. Serve at room temperatureor chilled. Enjoy!

# Challah Bread Pudding with Dried Cherries

*(Ready in about 35 minutes | Servings 6)*

### *Ingredients*

1. 7 slices challah, torn into bite-sized pieces

1. 3 tablespoons butter

1. 2 cups milk

1. 1 cup water

1. 4 eggs

1. 3 tablespoons rum

1. 1/2 teaspoon hazelnut extract

1. 1/2 teaspoon vanilla extract

1. A pinch of salt

1. 1/4 cup sugar

1. 1 tablespoon honey

1. 1/4 teaspoon grated nutmeg

1. 1/2 cup dried cherries

## Directions

1. Throw challah pieces in a lightly greased baking dish.

2. Next, make the custard by mixing all the remaining ingredients, except fordried cherries.

3. Pour custard mixture over challah. Now let challah absorb egg mixture.Scatter dried cherries over the top. Cover with an aluminum foil.

4. Lay trivet in the inner pot of your cooker. Pour in two cups water. Insert thebaking dish and lock the lid.

5. Select "Manual" function; set the timer to 25 minutes. Lastly, do a naturalpressure release. Serve at room temperature.

# Amazing Chocolate Cheesecake

*(Ready in about 1 hour | Servings 10)*

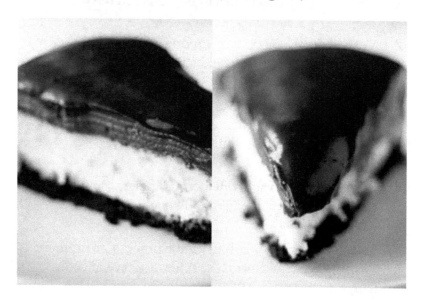

### *Ingredients*

For the Crust:

1. 1 ½ cups almond flour

1. 1/2 cup sugar

1. 1/4 cup coconut oil, room temperatureFor the Filling:

1. 1 ½ cups cashews, soaked and drained

1. 1 cup non-dairy milk

1. 1/2 cup non-dairy chocolate chips

1. 1 teaspoon vanilla essence

1. 1/4 teaspoon cinnamon powder

1. 1/2 teaspoon sea salt

1. 2/3 cups sugar

## *Directions*

1. Mix all the crust items. Press the crust mixture into a silicone cheesecakepan. Press with the back of a spoon and transfer to a refrigerator.

2. Then, make the filling by mixing all the filling items. Pour the filling overthe crust.

3. Put the trivet into the Instant Pot. Now lower the cheesecake pan onto thetrivet. Place IP lid on, and select "MANUAL"; cook for 55 minutes.

4. Afterwards, let pressure release naturally. Transfer the pan to a cooling rackbefore serving. Serve well chilled.

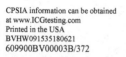

CPSIA information can be obtained
at www.ICGtesting.com
Printed in the USA
BVHW091535180621
609900BV00003B/372